ALAN E. SMITH

101

TIPS for
BETTER
and MORE
HEALTHY
SLEEP

Loving Healing Press

Ann Arbor, MI

D1720971

978-1-61599-717-6 paperback
978-1-61599-718-3 hardcover
978-1-61599-719-0 eBook

Loving Healing Press   www.LHPress.com
5145 Pontiac Trail   info@LHPress.com
Ann Arbor, MI 48105   Toll free 888-761-6268

Earlier works by Alan E Smith include *How To UnBreak Your Health* (www.unbreakyourhealth.com) and *101 Ways to Improve Your Health With Body Work*.

Contents

Solving Your Sleep Puzzle

All of your physical and mental health depends on getting a good night's sleep. We all love waking up without an alarm, feeling rested and refreshed, right? Unfortunately, many people don't sleep enough or sleep well, or both. There are almost as many reasons for not sleeping well as there are stars in the sky, or at least it seems that way some nights. You've probably tried a few things to sleep better that may or may not have worked for you. It may feel like your sleep is a combination lock and you can't figure out all the right numbers in the right sequence. These tips are designed to help you put it all together.

You have to adjust to factors outside your control that impact your sleep. An example is switching between daylight saving time and standard time. This has a many health effects like increased risk of heart attack and stroke. The U.S. Senate in 2022 passed a bill to make daylight savings time permanent, but the House stopped the bill, concerned that this is the wrong option. Many sleep experts say we should make standard time permanent, since it more closely follows sunlight. We all need sunlight in the morning to train our circadian rhythms to wake up and then fall asleep at night. This issue has yet to be resolved and it will affect everyone.

These 101 Tips are designed to help you find the rest you deserve in the best way possible. You'll walk through all of the various factors in getting a good night's sleep, from your bed and bedroom to relaxing before bed to solving several sleep problems. There are over the counter (OTC) drugs that can help, along with various supplements and herbs. While some of these tips have been around for hundreds or thousands of years, some are as new as they can be. Occasionally we talk about doctors and the progress that's been made in the medical field regarding sleep in past few decades.

Whatever your sleep situation, you will probably find something here that can help you sleep even better and longer. You just have to have the patience and dedication to solve your own sleep problems.

Sleep Basics

"There is a time for many words, and there is also a time for sleep."

— Homer, *The Odyssey*

Tip #1: Sleep Has Many Benefits

We need to accept that every human being needs to sleep every 24 hours, but even today scientists don't understand everything about sleep. We do know that sleep allows for both the body and the brain to repair themselves in critical ways and to restore energy. Sleep allows us to consolidate memories, handle information processing, aids our physical growth and muscle repair, along with countless other processes that are theorized to occur during sleep. We can't forget that sleep is also critical for strengthening our immune system and allowing us to fight off disease. We may not understand it all yet but we know that it is critical.

Tip #2: Sleep is Important to Brain Function

We don't need to know where sleep happens inside us, but having this information doesn't hurt. The *hypothalamus* is a small, peanut-sized structure deep inside the brain. It contains groups of nerve cells acting like control centers, which affect our sleep and waking. The brain stem is located at the base of the brain and it communicates with the hypothalamus. This controls the transitions between wakefulness and sleep.

Tip #3: Follow Your Personal Circadian Rhythm

Our bodies have a biological clock inside, which runs for a 24-hour day. This clock controls our circadian rhythm, which in turn controls a wide variety of functions. These synchronize with our environmental factors like light and temperature, but they continue even without those cues. They range from the daily fluctuations in wakefulness to body temperature, metabolism, and even the release of hormones. They control the timing of our sleep, meaning they cause you to be sleepy at night and awaken you in the morning, even without an alarm.

Tip #4: Your Sleep Needs Change Throughout Your Life

It varies depending on your own unique biological clock and your age. There isn't a simple answer, because we're all unique. Babies begin sleeping 16 to 18 hours each day (even if parents don't believe it). Their sleep needs change as they grow and their brains develop. School-age kids average over 9 hours of sleep each night, but the time they want to sleep shifts, with teens wanting to go to sleep later and rise later. Most adults need 7 – 9 hours of sleep every day, but after we turn 60, our sleep usually becomes shorter and lighter as we wake up several times each night.

Tip #5: Busting the "8 Hour" Myth

The simple answer is No. Our genes play a significant role in how much sleep we really need, along with our epigenetics or how our environment activates our genes. A recent report says that 1/3 of US adults usually get less than the recommended amount of sleep for one reason or another. Contributing factors include sleep environment, job or family stress, physical or mental health and many, many other variables. We do know that poor sleep can lead to obesity, diabetes and many other health problems. We all need to figure out and understand how much sleep works for our unique DNA. As part of your monitoring exercise, note how rested you feel at various times of the day.

Tip #6: There Are Sleep Minimalists

There are adults who simply need to sleep less due to their genes. It's estimated that 5% of Americans fall into this category. That means that they sleep normally 2 – 4 hours each night and yet are rested and refreshed when they wake up. It also means they have many more hours to work or play *every* day. Just imagine what you could accomplish if you had all of those extra hours each day! The important lesson here is never to compare your sleep needs to others. As Shakespeare said in *Much Ado About Nothing*: "Comparisons are odious".

Tip #7: There Are Consequences of Sleep Deprivation

Sleep deprivation has more serious consequences than just being more likely to be overweight. The weight issue is due to sleep affecting two appetite-controlling hormones, leptin and ghrelin. Leptin will signal to your brain that you've had enough to eat. When leptin levels are high, our appetite is reduced. Ghrelin does the opposite -- when ghrelin levels are high, you don't feel satisfied by the food you ate. It's been shown that people who are deprived of sleep have these two hormones go in opposite directions: there's a marked drop in leptin, which means an increase in appetite, while ghrelin rises, which leaves people unsatisfied.

More important than weight is the fact that folks who are frequently sleep deprived also have more strokes, cardiovascular disease, infections and even certain types of cancer than people who get enough sleep. This is especially important for people who work 2nd and 3rd shifts. These folks need all of the help they can get because 97% of them are never able to adjust their sleep cycle. The lesson here is simple: you can't cheat sleep – not in short term and especially not in the long term. Sleep is just as important as your other vital signs: respiration, temperature, blood pressure, and pulse.

Tip #8: Discover your Chronotype

You've heard the expression that someone is a "night owl" or perhaps an "early bird." This refers to their "chronotype" or an individual's preferred period for sleeping or being awake, which is due to their biologically programmed circadian rhythm. If you're a night owl, don't get a job on a dairy farm where the work starts at 4 a.m., or if you're an early bird don't work as an overnight ambulance dispatcher!

Tip #9: Melatonin and It's Role in the Sleep Cycle

People who have lost their sight and can't synchronize their sleep-wake cycle using natural light can often stabilize their sleep patterns by taking small amounts of melatonin at the same time each day. It's believed that the rise and fall of melatonin over time is critical for matching the body's circadian rhythm to the normal cycle of daytime and nighttime.

Before Going To Bed

"Man is a genius when he is dreaming."
— Akira Kurosawa

Tip #10: Obey the Most Obvious Sleep Signals

It sounds like a no-brainer but this tip is fundamental for a good night's sleep. If you only go to bed when you're getting sleepy, it will minimize the amount of time that you're awake in bed, which reinforces that being in bed means it's time to sleep.

Tip #11: Consistency is Key, So Establish a Baseline Schedule

As beneficial as all of these tips can be, it's important to remember that your body needs to know what to expect. In other words, you need to establish a consistent schedule and follow it every day or at least as closely as possible. There are folks who sleep in different ways, often called Biphasic Sleep when sleep is split between two main segments each day. Also called Segmented or Bimodal Sleep, it simply means you don't sleep through the night. In Spain, the daily siesta falls into this category. Whatever mode of sleep is most natural to you, stick to it. You'll find that you don't experience daytime sleepiness as much. To help you determine how consistent you are, you may want to note that in your sleep diary to monitor your sleep and what's impacting it.

Tip #12: Manage Your Child's Naptime According to Their Age

Establishing a consistent bedtime is most important for children. While the time they go to bed will change as they grow up, it's the consistency that's key. Parents often use bedtime stories or songs to help calm them down and transition to sleep. While babies sleep up to 18 hours every day, there are normally several naps scattered throughout the time period. The number of naps declines until around one year old there is only one nap per day. Once your child stops napping you'll need to adjust their bedtime to add in that extra hour. You'll notice that as your child passes their natural sleep window, they'll get a second wind as a result of hormones that are produced. Up to about 12 years of age, they may also have sleep terrors or sleep walking. One "trick" I've heard about involves using air freshener or even canned air (for cleaning computer keyboards) and spraying it under the bed and in the closet to get rid of monsters.

Tip #13: Easy Adjustments for Sleep Cycle Problems

It appears that bright light during the day can help reset the body's natural sleep cycle. It can be either natural or artificial light, but it needs to be bright. Roughly 30 minutes to an hour's worth of sunlight will do the trick. For folks waking up too early in the morning, the light exposure should be later in the day. If you're having trouble going to sleep at night, then your light exposure should be in the morning.

Tip #14: Avoid Common Sleep Distractions

Sleep hygiene is critically important to getting a good night's sleep. First of all, your bedroom should be for sleep or sex and nothing else. Anything else that you do in that room distracts your mind from its primary purpose, sleep. There should not be a television, stereo or telephone (even cell phone) in the bedroom. Studies have shown that children near a cell phone or TV in their room sleep almost 21 fewer minutes each night.

First of all, the room needs to be dark. That means you may need to use room-darkening window shades or perhaps wear a sleep mask to bed. As everything else, there is a wide range of sensitivity to light. While kids may want a nightlight, some adults can't sleep if there's any light in the bedroom. Remember, light is how we regulate our sleep, so be aware of its impact.

Tip #15: Control Your Sound Environment for the Best Sleep

Even if you live out in the country where it's relatively quiet, there's probably noise where you live. It could range from a quiet car driving by at night to the constant roar of living in the city with sirens, alarms and traffic all of the time. To minimize noise that can impact your sleep, you may need some type of white-noise device or fan, or even earplugs. There are white noise machines of every size and style, there are even headbands to deal with noise. They can play almost every sound imaginable from wind blowing through trees to waves on the beach. Remember, the bedroom you create is largely responsible for the quality of your sleep.

Tip #16: Getting Better Sleep On the Road

As challenging as it can be to find peace and quiet at home, it's much more difficult elsewhere. When you check into your hotel room, be sure to ask for a *quiet* room, away from the elevator, vending machines and ice machines. Check to be sure your room doesn't face a busy street or parking lot, too. Hopefully, the desk clerk will realize you don't want to be on the same floor or the floor below the visiting basketball team that likes to practice their dribbling.

Readjusting your sleep schedule in a new time zone can be very challenging, and the more time zones you've crossed the more difficult it can be, especially if you're travelling in an easterly direction. Jet lag not only means having difficulty sleeping but can also lead to diarrhea, headaches and other physical problems due to the changes in your circadian rhythm. First of all you'll want to take precautions for your trip by slowly adjusting your sleep schedule at home before you leave, and being sure to get plenty of sleep. Starting out tired only makes jet lag worse. Remember to drink plenty of water when you're in the air and at your destination, because dehydration also worsens jet lag.

If you're travelling more than eight time zones from home to the east, you'll want to wear sunglasses and avoid bright sunlight in the morning, but then get as much sunlight as possible in the late afternoon for the first few days. The reverse is true if you're travelling more than eight time zones to the west. You'll want to avoid sunlight a few hours before it gets dark locally for the first few days to help you adjust to your new location. Of course you'll want to remember other sleeping tips when you travel, too, like taking melatonin before bed.

Tip #17: Audio Meditations Can Help You Fall Asleep

Many folks need a little help going to sleep, so they use some type of sleep CD to help them drift off. A wide range of these products is available today from natural sounds to relaxing music to self-hypnosis to guided imagery or meditation, even bedtime stories for adults and kids. There are whole sleep CDs for adults and for children. You may want to experiment with different types of CDs to find what works best for you. A word of caution, if you're using a downloaded CD on your cell phone, be sure to set your phone's Do Not Disturb for a good night's rest. Systematic relaxation or some type of self-hypnosis can do wonders to help you fall asleep and to sleep better but it's a skill that you'll need to learn and practice.

Tip #18: Try Active Breath Control to Help You Fall Asleep

Yes, slowing your breathing down can help you relax, calm down and release stress. *Pranayama*, defined as breath control, is breathing exercises to control the flow of energy in your body. Normally done in a sitting position as part of a yoga routine, it can also be used to help you calm down and go to sleep. Simply breathe in through the nose, slow and steady, down into your stomach while letting go of all stressful or worrisome thoughts by concentrating on your breathing. Obviously, if you have any breathing or respiratory issues you'll need to consult with your doctor before beginning this sleep aid. There is a phone app also called Pranayama which you can try too.

Monitoring Your Zzzzs

"Truth, like love and sleep, resents approaches that are too intense."

— W. H. Auden

Tip #19: An Oura Ring Can Tell You About Your Sleep

There has been an amazing growth in technology to help you understand and hopefully improve your sleep. Have you heard of the Oura Ring? It's a ring packed with lots of technology to monitor your fitness, but also your sleep. For folks who don't want to wear a watch to bed, this little ring offers lots of information in a very small package that feeds an app on your smartphone, providing a wealth of information.

Tip #20: The Apple Watch Can Also Help

Yep, Apple not only makes computers but computers you wear. Heartbeat, blood oxygen, ECG and many other functions are available from this watch.

Tip #21: FitBit Trackers Now Monitor Sleep Time

Yes, the newer FitBit trackers, starting with Charge 4, features several sleep functions. In addition to heartbeat, breathing and blood oxygen levels, it also records your stages of sleep, even your snoring and the noise levels in your bedroom. All of this information can help you figure out your sleep problems for better sleep.

Tip #22: Smart Beds Know How You're Sleeping

For example, Sleep Number 360® beds come with SleepIQ® technology, which measures several key factors in how you're sleeping. The bed not only knows when you slept and for how long, but how well you slept and you don't have to wear anything because the technology is built into your bed.

Tip #23: Use Technology to Discover Your Sleep Stages

Lots of things! For example, sleep cycles are the range of the depth of your sleep, from Stage 1 very light sleep to Stage 5 deep sleep. In Stage 1 you're almost awake with normal breathing and almost normal muscle tone. Stage 2 is deeper sleep where you're less likely to be woken up, this is normally when REM sleep or dreaming takes place. Stages 3 and 4 are deep sleep, also called Slow Wave Sleep, where you're often difficult to awaken. Stage 5 sleep is the deepest part of your sleep cycle, and is its most restorative part.

Tip #24: Deep Sleep Is Very Important

Deep sleep is incredibly important, since this stage provides the most rejuvenating and restorative sleep. During deep sleep, your muscles repair and grow, your immune system is refreshed and your brain flushes out toxins. In addition, your blood pressure drops while your heartbeat and breathing rates are steady. While it usually occurs during the early part of your sleep, it can be up to 35% of your total sleep. Most adults spend 15% - 20% of their sleep in this stage. Sadly it decreases as you get older. You'll notice this is also the most difficult stage to wake up from. Use a sleep monitor, such as a smartwatch or fitness tracker, to find out how much deep sleep you're getting.

Tip #25: Making Sleep Efficiency Work for You

Sleep efficiency is simply the amount of time in minutes actually asleep divided by the amount of time in bed. Normal sleep efficiency should be 85% or higher. Most sleep technology (watches, rings, beds, etc.) measures sleep efficiency because it is a key indicator of the quality of your sleep and one which you may not be aware of because you think you're already asleep or that you were only awake for a few minutes in the middle of the night. You can start a "sleep journal" to correlate how your life activities and sleep hygiene affect your sleep efficiency.

Tip #26: Sleep Latency is the First Step

The first step toward deep sleep is measuring the time it takes you to fall asleep, called "sleep latency," and it is another key factor in understanding the quality of your sleep. A normal adult will fall asleep in 10 – 20 minutes. If you're falling asleep faster than that it may be because you're overly tired, or some other factor like alcohol. If it takes longer than 20 minutes to fall asleep or return to sleep, then there is probably another problem like stress, tomorrow's work, pain, exhaustion, caffeine or other issue that needs to be addressed.

Tip #27: How Quickly Should I Start To Dream?

Dreaming takes place in Rapid Eye Movement or REM sleep, so termed because your eyes will move quickly from one side to the other behind your closed eyelids. Normally, REM sleep happens about 90 minutes after you fall asleep and your breathing becomes faster and irregular while your heart rate and blood pressure rise to almost waking levels. REM sleep has several names like active sleep, desynchronized or paradoxical sleep and even rhombencephalic sleep. This stage is important because it's involved with brain development and emotional processing. If you sleep in sessions of shorter than 90 minutes, you won't reach REM sleep and this pushes you into sleep deprivation.

Tip #28 Restlessness Ruins Restfulness

Tossing and turning during sleep can make you feel tired during the day, like you didn't get a good night's sleep, because you didn't. Today's technology can measure Restfulness because it keeps track of excessive movement while you're asleep and how often you're getting up during your sleep. When you review your night's sleep results, does your movement happen due to snoring (yours or someone else's) or a pet on the bed? Does it happen at specific times of the night or in the early morning light? Keeping a sleep diary can help you figure out what's causing the problem, so you can improve the quality of your sleep.

Tip #29: Heart Rate Matters During Your Sleep Cycle

Several types of health technology can measure your heart rate, because it's of critical importance. Normal resting heart rates range from 60-80 beats per minute, but obviously your sleeping heart rate is even lower. Some types of health technology not only measure your lowest heart rate but also your average heart rate. They can even measure your heart rate variability, which can range between below 20 to over 120, and track it over time. HRV can also react to stress or illness before your resting heart rate. Monitoring the numbers and also the graphs of your heart can help you keep an eye on your sleep and your health.

Tip #30: Erasing A Sleep Debt

How big is your sleep debt or sleep deficit? Have you not been able to sleep for more than 24 hours or are you simply not getting enough sleep every night? Some estimates are that over 40 million Americans suffer from some amount of sleep deficit. What we do know is that not getting enough sleep can result in diminished physical and mental abilities like increased daytime sleepiness, poor concentration or short-term memory, even mood problems. Chronic sleep deprivation can result in more serious consequences like depression, weight gain and even diabetes. Fortunately, most short-term effects of sleep debt can be quickly reversed simply by getting enough sleep. Long-term effects will take much longer for recovery. If you wake up feeling tired even after enough hours of sleep, you may need to see a board-certified sleep doctor to discover the problem.

Designing Your Ideal Sleep Environment

"I had a dream I was awake and I woke up to find myself asleep."

— Stan Laurel

Tip #31: Buying a New Mattress Could Buy You Better Sleep

If your bed is 7 – 10 years old, it's probably time to invest in a new one. After all, you spend one-third of your life in bed! *Consumer Reports* lists 239 different mattresses from 81 different companies with prices ranging from $275 to $5,000. You have a choice from old-fashioned inner-spring mattresses and water beds to the latest mattress innovations of foam, gel, adjustable air or one of the many variations of hybrid mattresses. The first thing you need to do is determine exactly what your sleep requirements are so you can find the right mattress for your individual needs. Are you tall, medium or short? Do you sleep on your back, your side or your stomach? Do you normally enjoy a mattress that is firm, medium or soft? Those are some of the basic questions you need to answer before you go to a store. When you're shopping, remember to ask about the mattress's trial period, expected durability and warranty.

Tip #32: Your Mattress Matters More than You Think

Remember the children's story by Hans Christian Andersen about the princess who couldn't sleep because there were three peas under her huge pile of mattresses? It's a fanciful example of how little it takes for some people to have trouble sleeping and how important it is to choose the right mattress. It's especially important to remember when shopping for an innerspring or coil mattress. You probably recognize some of the bigger companies like Sealy, Serta, Sterns & Foster and Beautyrest.

This is perhaps the oldest basic style of mattress. They frequently have very little padding so the open springs allow air to circulate to prevent heat from building up. This also means the mattress uses the metal coils for their support. The amount of support depends on the gauge of the metal used, and how many springs are in the mattress. The lower the gauge number, the thicker the coil itself, resulting in a firmer feel. Some mattresses have different layers of springs or placement of springs that are made from different gauges of steel. Some encase their springs with fabric to stabilize their motion and muffle noise. Be sure to shop for firmer spring coils on the edge of the mattress for added durability.

Some of the newer innerspring mattresses do have additional padding, foam or even pillowtops above their springs. There is an almost endless variety of mattress types and combination of features for you to choose from. If you're concerned about motion transfer from a partner or pet, this may not be the best type of mattress for you.

Tip #33: Try a Different Type of Mattress

There is a wide range of foam and memory foam mattresses available today. This type of mattress shapes itself to your body, which provides outstanding pressure relief and support, so it's great for folks who suffer with aches and pains. You also won't feel motion from others moving on your mattress.

They come in a variety of foam types, shapes, thicknesses, densities and even combinations of foam. From egg crate to solid to open-air channels to other shapes of foam and memory foam, these mattresses offer a wide spectrum of options for you to find your best type of mattress. Some of the more popular brand names include Tempur-Pedic, Casper, Helix Midnight, Ghost Bed and Puffy. However be aware that this type of mattress will probably need to air out for at least 24 hours to reduce its chemical smell, called off-gassing.

Tip #34: Modern Air Mattresses are Not Just for Camping!

Most of us remember an air mattress as being something that you'd blow up to sleep on while camping. Today, air mattresses have come a long way. Now there are also air beds. Today an air mattress or bed can have one air chamber or several. They can allow you to have a firmer bed one night and a softer one the next time, depending on your aches and pains. Some can also be adjusted so partners can customize their side of the bed. SleepNumber brand beds even feature dynamic pressure relief and responsive air technology, meaning the bed adjusts to your movements during the night. Air mattresses can be noisier than other types of beds from their motorized parts pumping air or even from the air moving through their chambers. They also tend to retain body heat although some types of air mattresses have foam or gel layers to help with the heat issues. Some air mattresses also suffer from "trenching" or the gap between air chambers, which tends to sink under your weight. There's a lot to consider when shopping for an air mattress or an air bed. Some of the more popular brands of airbeds today are SleepNumber, Ghost Bed, Solaire, Puffy, Helix and ReST Bed.

Tip #35: Modern Waterbeds May Help

Most folks think that waterbeds began in the 1960s with the creation of vinyl, but the idea actually goes back hundreds, some say even thousands, of years. The first waterbeds in America were simply one giant bag of vinyl filled with water and heated from beneath. These waterbeds were comfortable for one person but challenging for two because of the wave motion of the water whenever one person moved. In the following decades, there have been design improvements with chambers and baffles to minimize the flow of the water. More recently, there have been hybrid waterbeds built with air and foam to maximize the benefits of water and minimize the problems. Today, there are hard-sided waterbeds that rest inside a wooden frame, and soft-sided versions that are water mattresses inside a foam frame. Both rest on a wooden base. Try a night on a waterbed and see for yourself.

Tip #36: Choose A Pillowtop Mattress For Extra Comfort

A pillowtop mattress is simply a mattress with an extra layer of padding on top for additional comfort, usually on an innerspring or memory foam mattress. They require less breaking in and offer less motion transfer than a regular mattress, but they also tend to trap heat and still require head/foot rotation. They also aren't recommended for heavier people.

Tip #37: Finding a Bed that Fits a Limited Space

Yes, there are options for limited space, for example a Trundle Bed. This is basically two twin beds, one stored underneath the other until it's needed, making it ideal for small living spaces. It works great in kids' bedrooms because it allows for sleepovers. These use a standard twin-sized mattress for the top bed and a slightly smaller mattress underneath.

Tip #38: Sofas that Transform Into Beds

There are different sizes and styles of sofa beds. This looks like a normal sofa during the day but at night you can remove the top cushions and pull a complete bed out. There are also sofa beds where the back of the sofa lies down, creating a bed. As usual, there is a variety of designs using different types of mattresses and springs. Whether as a primary sleep surface or just for guests, it's a very effective, space-saving type of furniture. They're also called a hide-a-bed or sleeper-sofa. These can be used to convert a living room into a temporary guest bedroom.

Tip #39: Is There A Difference Between a Sofa Bed and Day Bed?

These are frequently interchangeable terms describing the same type of furniture. While most sofas have a depth between 18 and 22 inches, a daybed normally uses a twin mattress which is 38 inches deep. However, if you throw a few pillows on the back to fill the space, it easily converts to a sofa. This is normally used in smaller living spaces.

Tip #40: Consider Other Space-Saving Types of Beds

A Murphy Bed or wall bed is a bed designed to be pulled down from the wall or closet. They come in a variety of sizes and can use different types of mattresses but normally memory foam or latex mattresses are best for this type of bed. (Don't try this with a waterbed!) The type of Murphy Bed is limited only by your imagination and design skills. The advantage of it is that when put away vertically during the day it opens up a great deal of living space.

Tip #41: Try a Japanese-style Futon Mattress

This is another type of mattress that became more popular in the 1960s, but it's actually a traditional type of Japanese bedding that is simply a cushion filled with cotton, leaves and sometimes even flowers. Part of its popularity is because it is relatively light and easy to fold and store in a closet during the day or move from room to room so it's great for small living conditions. It can also be used with a futon frame, which shapes the mattress like a couch during the day and can then be laid flat at night. While they usually only last up to five years, they are meant to be used on the floor or tatami and they do not provide a great deal of support or comfort. If you have a bad back, this probably isn't the mattress for you.

Tip #42: Consider a Hybrid Mattress

As you can already tell, several different types of mattresses can be combined to maximize their positive features and minimize the negative ones. Normally, a "hybrid" mattress is an addition on top of a normal innerspring mattress, but there are many different types of combinations. Does all of this make it harder to choose a mattress and bed? Absolutely! Just like your own individual genes and circadian rhythm, finding just the right type of bed and mattress depends on finding what works for you. Oh, and if that isn't hard enough, you have to remember there are also mattress toppers to consider, which can be memory foam, latex, air, organic (cotton and wool) and almost anything you can think of.

Tip #43: Discover the Right Pillow For You

For every type of variable and difference we've talked about for mattresses and beds, there are at least that many variations when we talk about pillows, maybe more. You want to be sure your head is hitting just the right kind of pillow for you. If you use pillows for your knees or back or any other body part, you'll want to also pay attention to that pillow. What size pillow do you want? What shape? There are standard, rectangular pillows, round, square, contour, boomerang, knee, body, lumbar, neck, wedge, horseshoe, travel and many other shapes. Then you'll need to choose the type of filling, beginning with the traditional feather and then moving through pillows filled with down, cotton, foam, shredded foam, multi-foam, latex, gel, polyfill, buckwheat, rice, water, microbeads, inflatable and many others. There even cooling pillows, pillows for pregnancy and pillows to use with a CPAP machine today. What kind of cover do you want for your pillows? Think this is complicated? You're just getting started! Make a list of the most important pillow attributes you want before you go shopping for that next great pillow.

Tip #44: Choose the Sheets that Make You Feel Great

Choosing the right kind of sheets to put on your new bed and mattress is almost as complicated as every other step in this process. First you need to be sure you're getting the right size of sheet for your mattress. Do you have a California King, King, Split King, Queen, Twin, Twin XL? Yes, you could choose cotton sheets but what kind of cotton? American, Egyptian, Long Staple or Supima? What about thread count? Lower thread counts tend to mean the sheets will feel rough. Higher thread count sheets may be softer and more comfortable but it also means there is less room between the threads for air to breathe so they can retain body heat. What type of weave in your cotton? Do you want percale, flannel, Sateen or Jersey? Or you want some other type of material like satin, silk, linen, polyester, bamboo, eucalyptus or microfiber? Remember you're trying to find the best environment for your best sleep so discover what makes you the most comfortable.

Tip #45: Try a Weighted Blanket for Psychological Comfort

Almost every variation in size and material we just talked about in sheets is also available as a blanket, with a few more additions like wool and fleece. There are additional options to consider, like do you want a weighted blanket? These are usually heavier than normal, which is said to offer a calming effect. Many times doctors will recommend a weighted blanket for individuals suffering from anxiety, restless legs or body, autism and such, since their deep pressure calms them down and improves the quality of their sleep. Or do you want an electric blanket to add some warmth on cooler nights? I'm not even going to go into bedspreads, quilts, duvets other coverings!

Tip #46: Pick the Right Clothes for Sleeping

Because comfort is your priority and there are lots of choices for men and women, starting with wearing nothing. After that, for men the options range from nightshirts to long-sleeved tops with long pants to short-sleeved with shorts to sleep or sweatpants or sleep shorts to hooded onesies to pajamas with feet, and of course they all come in a variety of fabrics from cotton to flannel to linen to silk or satin or a variety of synthetics. For women, there are even more options when you consider the variety of lingerie available in a world of fabrics and styles. Do you want to wear socks to bed? They're actually recommended to speed falling to sleep. What about a nightcap in the winter? Not a bad idea if your bedroom is very cool. Again, you need to determine what works best for you.

Sleep Lifestyle Makeover

"For in our dreams we find ourselves. Who we were. Who we are. Who we can become. Sleep. Dream."
— Moira Young, *Rebel Heart*

Tip #47: Exercise Can Help You To Sleep Better

Regular exercise helps both your brain and your body. Doctors don't know how or why exactly exercise helps you fall asleep faster and sleep better, but they do know it works. It may only take twenty or thirty minutes of exercise, but the question is the timing. There isn't a guaranteed "right" time of day to exercise for everyone, but it does appear that morning is a little better. But perhaps it's only a walk around the block after dinner. We do know that you shouldn't exercise anywhere close to bedtime. We also know that for those over 65 years of age, yoga and tai chi are best. Remember that you want to stretch before exercising and to use proper form, whatever type of exercise you choose.

Tip #48: Controlling Napping Is Important

In theory, napping is a good thing to help you recover from a poor night's sleep. In theory. The challenge is to limit yourself to a maximum of 30 minutes and to do it no later than 3 p.m., or the odds are you'll mess up your sleep at night. If you aren't careful, you can get into a cycle of longer, later naps interfering with your sleep at night, which requires more and longer naps.

Tip #49: Your Diet Affects Your Sleep

Research has shown that folks who eat a Mediterranean-style diet, meaning lots of fruits and vegetables, fish and whole grains, have a 35% lower risk of insomnia. They are also 1.4 times more likely to enjoy a good night's sleep. Don't go to bed hungry or overfull, because that will interfere with your sleep. You want to find your particular dietary sleep zone. Try to avoid heavy or large meals or spicy foods within a few hours of your normal bedtime.

Tip #50: Avoid Unnecessary Stimulants

OK, but only drink decaffeinated and keep that to a minimum, because there's still some caffeine left in it. You really need to avoid caffeine (and nicotine too) later in the day, because it's a stimulant to your nervous system. While it can give you a boost of energy and keep you awake, it can also give you insomnia, heartburn and increase your blood pressure. Remember that energy drinks are loaded with caffeine, so be careful with them too. Caffeine comes from more than 60 types of plants like coffee beans, tea leaves, kola nuts (think soft drinks) and cacao pods (think chocolate).

Tip #51: Alcohol Doesn't Help Sleep the Way You Think it Does

Appreciate that while a moderate amount of alcohol can help you relax and fall asleep more quickly, it will also have a negative impact on the duration and quality of your sleep, which will result in being more tired the following day. The effects of alcohol on sleep have been studied for decades, so we know that to be a fact. We also know that the effects of alcohol vary by the amount and speed of consumption along with the age, sex and physical shape of the person. Remember, the more alcohol you consume the more pronounced the effects. It's one thing to have a glass of wine with dinner, but something very different to have a bunch of margaritas before, during and after dinner.

Tip #52: Will Marijuana Help My Sleep?

Possibly. This seems to depend on your physical health and how often you use it. Folks suffering from chronic pain, PTSD, multiple sclerosis and even Restless Legs Syndrome report that weed helps them fall asleep faster, wake up less and have better quality sleep. However regular weed users are more likely to have sleep problems such as less sleep overall, slower to fall asleep and even less time in deep sleep. If you want to use marijuana as a sleep aid, you should probably use one that contains more THC than CBD.

Tip #53: Mom's Tip for Sleep Could Help You

How about a warm glass of milk to help you sleep? Yes, it's a very old-fashioned sleep aid that you probably heard about from your grandmother, since it's been passed down through the generations. The reason it's still around today is that it does seem to help, primarily due to at least two of its components, namely tryptophan and melatonin. Scientific studies show that it's especially helpful for those over 65 years old.

Does it really make a difference if it's warm or cold? It doesn't appear so, but warm milk may subconsciously remind us of being breast-fed as babies, so maybe it's slightly more beneficial. It's really up to your individual preference. You can also add flavor to your warm milk with sugar, honey, cinnamon, maple syrup, strawberries, bananas or even turmeric.

Tip #54: Avoid Eating Simple Carbs Just Before Bedtime

You're going to want simple or fast carbohydrates as bedtime snacks, which are carbs that break down and burn more quickly in your body, which will help you relax. Foods like fruits and nuts, milk and cheese, and some vegetables contain simple carbs as does rice, cake and candy. Foods such as bananas, mangoes and raisins have additional health benefits. However, be careful not to eat too much of these simple carbs too close to bedtime.

Tip #55: Chamomile Tea Will Help You Sleep

One ancient and reliable way to prepare for bed is with a cup of Chamomile Tea. Be careful when you first try this though, since people with allergies may be sensitive to chamomile. This traditional, caffeine-free folk remedy has been around for centuries. Today we know that it's loaded with antioxidants. It will calm you down and help you to relax, so you can fall asleep faster and sleep better. It's also reported to be beneficial for treating everything from menstrual cramps to cancer.

Tip #56: How to Unwind Before Bedtime

First of all, you shouldn't get all wound up right before trying to go to bed, you're trying to *unwind* and relax. That means no exciting or scary TV shows, no horror or thriller movies. It's no secret that children need limits on how much time they watch TV, especially near bedtime. Additionally, no more news programs that get you all pissed-off at the state of the country and/or world. Pumping a bunch of adrenaline into your system is just going to keep you awake. Instead you should be reading or watching something pleasant and not-work related. Listening to pleasant, easy music may help, too. If you have to watch TV in the evening, then stream an old sitcom from the '60s, '70s or '80s. You want your mind to be in a safe and happy place before bed.

Tip #57: Prayers or Affirmations Can Help You Unwind

Absolutely! Instead of trying to control or force sleep, it's much better to simply relax and let sleep find you. One of the ways to relax and unwind is to release all of the stress of the day to find your own calm. Do you have to pray the same prayer from your childhood? Only if you want to. There are many, many more prayer options today. You don't even have to pray to whatever God you choose, it can simply be a positive affirmation. Is all of this just mumbo-jumbo? No. The *Harvard's Medical Guide to a Good Night's Sleep* even suggests bedtime meditation because it calms your mind. As with other techniques, it would helps to practice this at least several times per week to get started.

Tip #58: How Can I Possibly Relax Before Bedtime After The Day I've Had?

This is one of the key issues for people having trouble going to sleep or staying asleep. One of the first steps is to "release the day" so it doesn't haunt your subconscious mind and ruin your sleep. One way to do this is to simply review and release all of the issues and/or problems of your day in reverse order to acknowledge them and put them on the shelf until tomorrow. It's harder than it sounds and it takes practice.

Another way to get rid of the day's stresses is to describe to yourself in your mind in a low, soft monotone the stressful or disturbing images you see from the day. Don't worry about how or why the images change, just acknowledge to yourself what you're seeing, that's what's important. The goal is to release the day.

Tip #59: Try Sleeping On It

You can take it one step further and use the time before sleep to actually help solve the problems you're having during the day. You've heard the old expression to just "sleep on it" to avoid making a rash or wrong decision? We've all had the experience of waking up with the solution to a problem, but did you know you can actually program your subconscious mind? You can put a request to your powerful subconscious mind for help, but only on one issue per night. This request must also be in positive terms like "I want to be slim" instead of "I don't want to be fat." Simply repeat this several times as you're falling asleep and it will help you relax and fall asleep.

Tip #60: What If I Have An Idea Or Solution In The Middle of The Night?

The easiest way to deal with this problem of your subconscious working too hard or too fast is to put a pad of paper and a pen or pencil next to your bed. That way if you do happen to wake up in the middle of the night you can simply write it down so you don't have to worry about losing it when you go back to sleep. By writing it down, you free yourself from the fear of losing it so you can relax and return to sleep.

Tip #61: Avoid Checking Your Phone Before Bedtime

You shouldn't have even looked at your cell phone so late in the day! For your own health and vitality, you need a good night's sleep and for that you need to be able to relax and unwind. Getting upset from an email isn't going to help you soon before bedtime. Besides, looking at a blue-light emitting device like a cell phone is known to disrupt our normal sleep patterns. To be your best, you need to sleep well, so turn on/set the Do Not Disturb function on your phone.

Tip #62: My Mind Is Relaxing, But My Body Is Still Stressed

How about a warm bath? (Bubbles or essential oils are optional.) This doesn't have to be more than ten minutes one to two hours before bed, but it can make a world of difference. First, it's very relaxing mentally and physically. Second, it tells the brain it's time to produce melatonin. Third, it drops your body's core temperature by moving more blood to your hands and feet. You might even consider adding a little soft music to help your relaxation.

Tip #63: Do I Have Insomnia?

Basically, if you haven't fallen asleep with 20 minutes or so, it's time to get out of bed and do something relaxing for either your mind or body or both. How about reading a book (sorry, no Stephen King novels)? Or listening to soothing music (no hard rock). Try a hypnotic meditation track, these are designed to help you relax and slow your breath into a sleep state. You need to try and resolve your worries before bed, so write down what's bothering you and then set it aside for tomorrow so you can relax and go to sleep.

Alternative Options

"As important as it is to have a plan for doing work, it is perhaps more important to have a plan for rest, relaxation, self-care, and sleep."

— Akiroq Brost

Tip #64: There Are Lots of Options To Help You Sleep

Yes, there are lots of options. You'll just need to discover which one(s) work best and most safely for you. Melatonin is the first tip, since it's the hormone that naturally increases about two hours before your normal bedtime and tells your brain that it's time to sleep. It's been studied since it's discovery in the 1950s. This over-the-counter product normally ranges from 1 mg to 10 mg and comes in about every form imaginable from tablets and capsules to liquid and sublingual. Be careful to look for USP Verified on the package. As with anything that you put into your body, there can be side effects, the most common with melatonin being headache, dizziness and nausea. There can also be feelings of depression, confusion or anxiety or even abdominal cramps. While abnormally low blood pressure is another side effect for those folks taking certain blood pressure medications, increased blood pressure is also possible. There can also be allergic reactions such as a skin rash, itching or more serious ones like swelling of the face, lips or tongue. You should always check with your doctor before you start putting anything new into your body. In response to a recommendation for prescription medication, simply say you want to try natural options first.

Tip #65: There Is Also GABA

Obviously another popular option is GABA, an amino acid and neurotransmitter responsible for slowing signals from one nerve cell to another. This produces a calming effect. There is a variety of opinions about it, including doubt that it can even get into your brain, through what's called the blood-brain barrier. Some say that GABA can't be found in foods but others say it can. Foods like spinach, sweet potatoes, broccoli, kale, brown rice, beans, chestnuts, mushrooms, tomatoes, cauliflower, Brussels sprouts are reported to contain GABA or boost its production in your body. It can also be found in some fermented foods like kimchi and miso, and in varieties of teas like green, black and oolong. GABA is also available in pill, capsule and even powder form. As with other supplements, the risk of side effects increases as dosage increases.

Tip #66: Aromatherapy with Lavender

One of the oldest treatments to improve your sleep is lavender. Ancient Greeks and Romans used lavender for a variety of purposes including as a treatment for insomnia. It's been proven to improve your body's melatonin levels, which you know are important to tell the brain it's time to sleep. It can also calm your nervous system. Lavender plants come in four different categories and can grow to between nine inches and three feet. Best of all, lavender is available without a prescription and it comes in many different forms so it's very easy to use. There's lavender soap for your bath, you can mix it with distilled water to make a spray for your bedroom or pillow, you can put it into a sachet or potpourri bag to put into your pillow or you can even make a tea with it. Be careful if you choose to use lavender essential oil. Mix it with other oils if you're going to apply it directly to your skin as a massage oil. It can also be used in a diffuser or you can use a lavender cream or salve.

Tip #67: Try Valerian Root Derivatives to Help Your Sleep

There are lots of supplements and treatments to help you fall asleep and sleep better. One that's been studied for almost four decades is Valerian root, a tall, flowering grassland plant that's even been shown effective for insomniacs, and that the European Medicines Agency has approved for sleep and anxiety since 2016. The effects aren't quick however. It seems to take from thirty minutes up to two hours to begin. There are Valerian root pills ranging from 300 to 600 milligrams, or you can make a tea with two to three grams of the dried root steeped for ten to fifteen minutes. The longer you brew it, the more intense the flavor will be, which folks describe as "woodsy," to something not as pleasant. You can also use Valerian essential oil in a diffuser as aromatherapy. Side effects with Valerian are similar to other sleep supplements ranging from headache and upset stomach to dry mouth and even vivid dreams.

Tip #68: Try Some Passionflower to Prevent Insomnia

Yes, Passionflower or *Passiflora incarnata* has been used for hundreds of years as a medicine. One of its uses is to reduce anxiety and aid sleep and insomnia by increasing the levels of GABA in your brain. However, research into the effectiveness of Passionflower varies from study to study. You can take a Passionflower capsule, use a 1:5 tincture once in the evening or enjoy a cup of tea that's been steeped for up to 20 minutes in the evening.

Tip #69: Lemon Balm Can Help You Sleep

Once again it's been used safely for hundreds of years to treat nervous stomach, digestive tract problems and insomnia. In fact, Carmelite nuns used to make an alcoholic tonic with lemon balm back in the 14th century. This is a plant in the mint family named for its lemony scent that helps calm people down so they can relax and go to sleep. It's available in capsule form, a tincture or you can brew a tea by pouring a cup of boiling water over 2-3 teaspoons of the dried herb and allowing it to brew for up to 15 minutes.

Tip #70: Hops To A Sleep Aid

OK, how about hops? Yes, we're talking about one of the main ingredients of beer. Its medicinal properties have been known since the ninth century. The sedative effects of hops was discovered almost by accident when field workers kept falling asleep on the job. Hops enhance GABA levels, but they also lower the body's core temperature, which is important to calm the nervous system and lower anxiety so you can fall asleep. Hops may be even more effective when combined with valerian. It comes in capsules, tincture or powder forms and you can even make a pouch of hops to breathe in the scent, a trick reportedly used by King George III. Simply put some dried hops into a pouch and put it into your pillowcase. You can even add lavender or passionflower to the mixture. Hops can even be made into a tea, but only brew it for 3 minutes. Some honey may help offset its bitter taste. A word of caution on hops, you'll want to stop using it at least two weeks before surgery and avoid it when drinking alcohol or taking sleeping pills. Hops should also be avoided by people with depression or where it would worsen symptoms.

Tip #71: Try an Ayurvedic Approach

Ashwaganda comes from the roots of Withania somnifera, part of the nightshade family, and is also known as Indian ginseng and winter cherry. It's been used for hundreds of years as part of traditional Ayurveda practices. It's been shown to be effective in helping people fall asleep faster, spend more time asleep and even enjoy better sleep quality. It comes in a variety of forms including powder, pill, tincture, tea and even gummies. The most common side effects include diarrhea, nausea, and vomiting. In addition there are less frequent side effects which include dry mouth, vertigo, hallucinations, blurred vision, rash and weight gain. While it appears that it can be taken for up to three months, there is evidence that it can cause liver damage.

Tip #72: Sage Smudging Improves Sleep, Too

Sage is a natural sedative with a long history of use in alternative and traditional medicine. It's an herb similar to basil, rosemary and oregano that's used in food around the world. Smudging is the ancient practice of burning sage, which can produce a sense of calm similar to meditation. Be careful though, because anyone with asthma or respiratory problems can have trouble with this, even cats. Sage can be used as an aromatic tea similar to mint. It's also available in pills and as an essential oil that can be inhaled with a diffuser, rubbed on the skin or by ingestion. Caution should be used with sage when taken in higher does for a long time.

Tip #73: Keep Some Kava Around For Better Sleep

Another supplement that seems to be effective at treating insomnia is kava or kava kava, a plant native to the South Pacific. The main effect appears to come from how it impacts the GABA neurons in the brain. Since this helps regulate the nervous system, kava helps you relax your muscles, calms the mind and helps you to stay in deeper stages of sleep longer. There are kava pills and capsules or kava tea, but the dosage can vary widely, so start with a low dose and build until it's effective for you.

Tip #74: Try American Skullcap

Skullcap is a flowering perennial plant in the mint family that the British Herbal Pharmacopoeia lists as a mild sedative. It has a long history as a sleep aid because it helps relax the body and mind. It should not be confused with Chinese skullcap, which is a different plant with different health benefits. It comes in capsule form ranging from 100 – 1200 mg but normal doses range between 350 – 1000 mg at bedtime. It can also be taken as a tea with a slightly bitter taste, or in tincture form. As with all supplements, use with caution and if you experience any side effects or discomfort, contact your physician.

Tip #75: Try Sacred Basil or Tulsi

How about Holy Basil? It's been called the "elixir of life" in ancient texts of Ayurveda and used in medicine for literally hundreds of years. You may also see it described as Sacred Basil or Tulsi. It's also been called "hot basil" due to its peppery taste so, clearly this isn't the spice your mom puts in her marinara sauce. Holy Basil has been used to treat a variety of health problems like nausea, bronchitis and even bug bites, but it's also a powerful herb for dealing with sleep disorders. This plant acts as an adaptogen, which means that it can help your body adapt to stress and reduce anxiety, allowing you to sleep better. It's recommended that you take it after the evening meal for better sleep, and it comes in several forms including powder, extract and oil. As with all supplements, the Food and Drug Administration (FDA) does not review their safety or effectiveness, so it is Buyer Beware.

Tip #76: Consider Wild Lettuce

There is also Wild Lettuce, which has been shown to be effective to help sleep for hundreds of years all over the world. It's also been called prickly lettuce, bitter lettuce, tall lettuce and even opium lettuce. There are even research studies that go back to the early 1800s. The plant contains lactucarium, which is a milky fluid that has both analgesic and sedative properties so it soothes nerves and pain and relieves mild insomnia symptoms. Wild lettuce is available in capsules, as an extract, a tincture or as a tea. Since it has minimal side effects, it's also commonly used in homeopathic sleep remedies. It can be toxic in higher doses, however. There are also reports of side effects, so if you suffer from narrow-angle glaucoma or an enlarged prostate you should be extremely careful and perhaps avoid this supplement. You may also suffer nausea, dizziness and sensitivity to light, sweating and even heart and breathing problems.

Tip #77: Sleep Like Your Grandmother Did

Another sleep aid you may have heard about from your grandmother is to eat or drink tart cherries an hour or two before bed. The reason this remedy has been passed down generation to generation is because it's been shown to help people sleep more and with better sleep quality. Two of the most common varieties of tart cherries are Montmorency and Balaton. These are different from the sweet cherries you may eat or cook with, so pay close attention. If you're going to use tart cherry juice, be sure to get unsweetened, without added sugar. You can also find it as an extract, capsules, frozen, dried or concentrated. Tart cherries may have a positive effect on your sleep due to two of its chemicals, melatonin and tryptophan, which we've talked about before. This can even help you get over jet lag when you travel. People who regularly take blood thinners should probably discuss adding tart cherries to their diet with their doctor.

Tip # 78: Try St. John's Wort

Another herbal supplement that may help you sleep better is St. John's Wort, which has also been used for centuries to treat depression and anxiety. It appears to stimulate the GABA receptor, and by increasing the production of melatonin, both of which are important to sleep, especially deep sleep. It may even help women reduce their hot flashes at night. It's available in capsules or pills, in tinctures and as a tea. The most common side effects are dizziness, diarrhea, dry mouth, headache and fatigue. Strangely enough, St. John's Wort may also increase your blood pressure when you consume foods high in tyramine such as sausage, salami, dried meats, cheeses, sauerkraut, red wine and beer. If you're taking antidepressants, use extreme caution since this can lead to serotonin syndrome. Also if you're taking Warfarin, St. John's Wort may increase the risk of blood clots.

Tip #79: Tapping Can Also Help Your Sleep

You may have already heard about EFT, or "tapping" as it's known, but did you know it can help you sleep? In the 1990s Gary Craig synthesized Thought Field Therapy (TFT), adding some NLP (Neurolinguistic Programming) concepts into a simplified form called

EFT or Emotional Freedom Techniques. By focusing on a problem like poor sleep or not being able to fall asleep while you tap on certain acupuncture points to stimulate them, you can change your mind and body. Since its creation, many improvements and variations have been created but this simple technique is easy to learn and perform, even while you're in bed.

Tip #80: NIH Says Acupuncture or Acupressure Can Help You Sleep

Would you believe that in 1997 the National Institutes of Health (NIH) endorsed the safety and effectiveness of acupuncture for treating sleep-related disorders like insomnia? Traditional Chinese Medicine has been around for thousands of years, so even if modern medicine doesn't understand it, this is a viable sleep aid. If you don't have access to an acupuncturist, you can stimulate the acupoints yourself without needles.

Begin by finding a comfortable position, take a few deep breaths to relax and then use deep, firm finger pressure. Start by pressing on the HT 7 Shenmen points, one being on the wrist just below the hand and the other on the edge of the little finger. Another popular treatment point is GB 20, GV20 or Baihui, which is at the highest point of the head in the center of the line between the tips of the ears. Located on the bottom of your foot is the K11 or Yongquan acupoint, which you can find in the small depression that appears in the small depression that is just above the center of your foot when you curl your toes. Whether stimulated by acupuncture or acupressure, these points will help balance your chi for better sleep. You can find posters or videos with these points demonstrated on Google.

Waking Up Before You're Ready

"Sleep's what we need. It produces an emptiness in us
into which sooner or later energies flow."
— John Cage, M: *Writings '67-'72*

Tip #81: Nothing Seems To Help, What About Taking A Pill?

There are sleep medications you can buy without a prescription that
are generally safe but may come with some risks. The most popular are
ZzzQuil and Sominex, which contain Doxylamine, is a sedating
antihistamine. You may also want to try Avinol PM Extra Strength,
SleepMD, Nytol or SimplySleep. If you want to go this route you'll
want to start with a low dose and also limit your alcohol intake,
because it can increase the sedative effects. Consult your doctor before
using any of these for longer than 3 consecutive weeks.

Tip #82: Lots of Over-The-Counter Medications Can Make You Sleepy

Many OTC medications contain pseudoephedrine, which can make
you sleepy but can also cause insomnia. This drug is in so many
products that a complete list would almost be a book by itself, but also
recognize that there's a reason it's stored behind the pharmacy counter,
even though you don't need a prescription for most of them.
Pseudoephedrine is a decongestant that will shrink blood vessels in
your nasal passages to relieve sinus congestion. You'll find this drug in
Actifed, Advil Cold & Sinus, Claritan-D, Contac Non-Drowsy,
Dimetapp Sinus, Dristan Sinus Maximum Strength Tylenol Sinus,
Sudafed and many other products. Don't use any of these products if
you have used an Monoamine oxidase inhibitor within the past 14
days, because a dangerous drug interaction can occur.

Tip #83: Your Pain Prevents You From Sleeping

Are you thinking about taking an Advil PM, Aleve PM, Bayer
PM, Excedrin PM or a Tylenol PM? These are just some of the over-
the-counter pills available to help you sleep. Most of them contain

Diphenhydramine (DPH) as their main ingredient, because the drug companies discovered that folks taking Benadryl complained about being sleepy or drowsy. Check the labels of whatever OTC pain or sleep aid you're interested in for its ingredients. Whenever you take this type of product, be very careful driving or operating machinery and use alcohol cautiously. There also appears to be a link between the use of this type of product and dementia, Alzheimer's, along with long-term liver damage and other issues.

Tip #84: What About Prescription Sleeping Pills?

If there's an event in your life disturbing your sleep like a divorce or death in the family, then a prescription sleeping pill may be a short-term solution. Realize that there are studies showing that they really aren't that beneficial: you might only get to sleep eight to twenty minutes sooner and you may suffer a hangover effect the next day as reported by eighty percent of study participants. You may also experience parasomnia, which can cause you to sleepwalk or even drive, eat, talk or even take medications and not remember anything after you wake up. Older folks are also more than five times more likely to experience an amnesiac effect like forgetfulness, confusion or dizziness.

There are several different prescription sleeping pills, but most are either antidepressants, Benzodiazepines or Z-drugs like Ambien® and Lunesta®. Other prescription sleeping aid brand names include Silenor, Rozerem, Restoril, Halcion, Ambien CR and Belsomra. You are going to need a doctor's prescription for this type of sleeping aid.

You will also need to be monitored by your physician to be sure you don't become addicted to them and to help you withdraw from their use. It can take several weeks or longer to get off of these medications. Also never mix alcohol and sleeping pills, ever.

Tip #85: My Doctor Says To Do A Sleep Study First

That's actually a good idea to determine what kind of sleep problems you're having in order to prescribe the correct medication. A sleep study or polysomnography can help diagnose a variety of sleep disorders like sleep apnea, restless legs syndrome, narcolepsy, sleep-walking, insomnia and more. Most sleep studies are done at a sleep center or hospital, but there are now home test devices for some sleep problems. Basically, you check into the facility in the evening and they wire you up with lots of electrodes to measure how you're sleeping, when you're sleeping, how you're breathing and many other vital elements of sleep. Overnight technicians monitor all of your sensors to watch for any problems and make notes for the doctor to review in the morning. This can be a very useful first step to solving your sleep problems.

Tip #86: My Doctor Won't Admit My Prescriptions Are Causing My Insomnia And Maybe More Problems

That's not uncommon, it's called drug-induced insomnia and it can be caused by everything from prescription asthma inhalers to steroids. One list of these problem medications has over 75 listings and it isn't even a complete list. A drug for high blood pressure, amlodipine, is one of the many known drugs to cause insomnia. Even over-the-counter medications can be the source of your insomnia. You're going to have to ask your doctor(s) specific questions about this and probably do some Internet research on your own so you'll know when you're being dismissed because the doctor is too busy. It's helpful just to be aware that this may be part of your sleep problems.

Tip #87: So Why Am I Always Sleepy Even If I'm Sleeping OK?

Feeling like you've been drugged isn't uncommon for many folks. This is the flip side to prescription drugs causing insomnia. Have you ever had surgery where you were given anesthesia? Then you know it can take days, weeks, even months to finally get all of those chemicals out of your system so you can sleep normally and be wide awake all day. Drugs can produce the same kind of sleep hangover, which is one of the many reasons you need to do your research before you start taking any type of sleep aid, even over the counter medications. You'll always want to start with the lowest dose possible and slowly work you way up to the right dosage for you. Don't just accept whatever your doctor prescribes, question why that particular drug and why that particular dose? Can you start with a lower dose? What are the side effects? How will it interact with your current medications? It's your body and it's unique so you need to be careful with it.

Tip #88: I Go To Sleep Fine But Wake Up In The Middle of The Night

Many folks wake up once or twice each night, but being *wide* awake and unable to go back to sleep is a different problem. Recognize that waking up between 1 a.m. and 4 a.m. and then not falling back to sleep is a symptom of what's called middle insomnia. If you can't go back to sleep in about 20 minutes, it may be time to get up and sit in a comfortable chair in another room before you return to bed to try again. Perhaps you should take another melatonin tablet? There are lower doses of melatonin marketed as "3 a.m." and "Midnight" versions. Do you have pain? Then you're going to probably need a pain reliever with PM in its name. Digestive problems like acid reflux or irritable bowel syndrome? You'll have to take care of it before you have a chance of returning to sleep.

One way to calm your body down so you can relax and return to sleep is a yoga technique called "progressive relaxation" where you gently tense each muscle and then relax it, beginning at your feet and slowly moving up your body. Another method of relaxation if you woke up from REM sleep and are able to remember the thoughts or dreams that you were having is to use the Theater of the Mind technique to first see what your subconscious wants you to see and then simply draw the curtains closed and return to sleep. You can find free progressive relaxation videos on YouTube or have your partner record one just for you.

Tip #89: Take Control of Nightmares

Would you believe that modern medical science doesn't really know why you dream? Most folks dream about two hours every night, but we don't remember most of them. Dreams are strongest during our REM sleep, when you're less likely to remember your dream. They may be a way of confronting emotional dramas in your life so your brain can make connections regarding your feelings that your conscious mind wouldn't make.

Moving up the scale a little is lucid dreaming, which is a dream where you know that you're actually dreaming. This usually happens between REM sleep and being awake. The good news is, some lucid dreamers are able to influence their own dreams to literally change the story. This is especially beneficial if you're experiencing nightmares. Further up the scale, the American Sleep Association says that about 5% of adults experience persistent nightmares while between one-half to two-thirds of children experience weekly nightmares. Many things can cause nightmares including stress, anxiety and many different types of medications including antidepressants, blood pressure drugs, and allergy medications. In some cases these nightmares become night terrors where the person may not wake up during them but instead will scream, cry or thrash around the bed.

One way to deal with these dreams is called Imagery Rehearsal Therapy or IRT, a type of cognitive-behavioral therapy that reduces the stress that occurs with recurrent nightmares. Simply put, you take a particularly scary image from the nightmare and then mentally restructure the image so it's no longer frightening or you put it into a less scary story and rehearse that story a few times.

Another way to deal with bad dreams is a Native American dream catcher. Believing that the night air is filled with good and bad dreams, they make a dream catcher to hang over or near the bed. Good dreams know how to pass through it and slide down the feathers while bad dreams get tangled in the dream catcher and disappear in the first light of the day.

Dealing with nightmares or night terrors with children needs a different solution since they completely trust their parents to keep them safe and kill their monsters. Adults can explain to the child that their parents used magic weapons or tools to get rid of them. Then they can spray monster-killing air underneath the child's bed and into their closet. This spray can be compressed air used to clean computers or even lavender air freshener, so long as this is the only use for this spray.

Sleeping With a Partner

"Sleep crawled on top of me like an affectionate, purring pet-"

— M.L. Rio, *If We Were Villains*

Tip #90: Why Do Old Men Go To The Bathroom So Often At Night?

It's not uncommon for men over the age of 50 to experience an enlarged prostate or benign prostatic hyperplasia (BPH for short), which causes them to make several trips to the bathroom every night. Yes, that makes it very difficult to get a decent night's sleep! Treatment options will depend on the patient's age, health status, severity of symptoms and the degree of enlargement of the prostate. In the most severe cases, surgical intervention may be required or at least prescription medications. However the good news is there are many over-the-counter options that will help this problem. The key ingredients in most of the OTC products are Beta Sitosterol, Pygeum, Saw Palmetto, Pumpkin seeds, Nettle, Zinc and Green Tea. They come in almost every possible combination of ingredients. Just a few of the brand names include: Prostara, Prostate Plus, 1MD Prostate MD, PureNature Prostafen, Puritan's Pride Saw Palmetto, Prostanol, VigRX Support, OptiProstate XTS, Urinozinc Prostate Plus, Prost8 Plus and Prostalieve.

Tip #91: Menopausal Women Need Help To Sleep Better

The most common problem of menopause is hot flashes, which is the feeling of extreme warmth in the upper body. When they happen at night they're called night sweats, which interrupt sleep. Modern medicine doesn't know why hot flashes happen but they're unique to each woman. While about 20% of women never get hot flashes or experience them only for a short period of time, the average experience seems to be about seven years. They can last for different amounts of time and vary in intensity. For some women it's a mild inconvenience, but for others it can be intense heat that impacts their life. There are many different triggers for hot flashes, ranging from hot weather to smoking or caffeine to stress or just about anything. Fortunately there are ways to deal with them, beginning with maintaining a healthy weight. Overweight women can experience more frequent and severe hot flashes. You can also dress in layers of lightweight, loose clothing made from natural fibers like cotton that can be easily removed when a hot flash strikes, although that isn't easy at bedtime. You could also try soy isoflavones, which bind to estrogen receptors and can help reduce hot flashes and night sweats. Or you could try black cohosh which is a very popular treatment that comes in capsules or tea. If you're having serious problems with hot flashes and night sweats, talk with your doctor about hormone replacement therapy or HRT for a limited time, usually less than five years.

Tip #92: Sleeping While Pregnant Can Be A Challenge

Sleep is naturally an essential part of prenatal care, but if you're having trouble sleeping well, recognize that it's not uncommon. A few of the more frequent sleep disorders during pregnancy are obstructive sleep apnea, Restless Legs Syndrome and gastroesophageal reflux disorder (GERD). Doctors normally recommend sleeping on your side during pregnancy, preferably on your left side, but there doesn't seem to be any research to determine whether the right or left side is best so feel free to switch back and forth. Sleeping on your left side also takes the pressure off your liver and kidneys, which may help with the swelling in your hands, ankles and feet. The main thing is to not sleep on your back, especially after the 28th week, because that does seem to carry risks for your child. In other words, you should sleep on your side keeping your legs and knees bent using pillows as necessary. (Check the Pillow Tip, too.)

Tip #93: Bedwetting for Young and Old

Let's start with a problem that affects both young and old, wetting the bed, also called nighttime incontinence or nocturnal enuresis, which is involuntary urination while asleep. For a small number of children, bed-wetting after age 7 can still be a problem. While no one knows for sure what causes bed-wetting, there are several issues that may be involved including a small bladder, an inability to recognize a full bladder, a hormone imbalance, or urinary tract infection. In some children going through a major life change like moving, or a new sibling can cause them to wet the bed again after being dry for ages. To help kids learn not to wet the bed, you can reduce drinks before bedtime and eliminate caffeinated drinks. Also you should encourage kids to use the bathroom 15 minutes before bed and again right before going to bed. Keep track of the nights they don't wet the bed and reward them, but never punish them for wetting the bed.

For adults, sleep apnea or diabetes may also be a factor in wetting the bed along with an enlarged prostate or an obstruction in part of the urinary tract from a bladder or kidney stone. Obviously, a medical exam is recommended when the bed-wetting occurs in an adult.

In either case, there are also new options to help with this problem. Today there are bed-wetting alarms for kids of all ages, which will wake them up so they can go to the bathroom and finish peeing. There are a variety of alarms ranging from sensor pads that go under the sheet to wearable ones. There are also diapers that can be worn to bed, which won't stop the problem but it will keep the bed dry. There are also waterproof sheets, which will also keep the mattress dry. Once the bed-wetting problem is resolved, you'll be able to sleep much better.

Tip #94: Other Suggestions To Help You Sleep

Of course! How about Cognitive Behavioral Therapy or CBT? This is a type of short-term talk therapy or psychotherapy where you work with a therapist in a limited number of sessions. It's been proven effective in treating insomnia and many other problems by helping you become aware of inaccurate or negative thoughts so you can respond in a more effective manner. For example, you can learn to identify negative thoughts or feelings and then to practice new skills in a real-world situation to solve problems in a better way. It would be one way to discover the source of your insomnia in order to deal with it more effectively.

There are also devices that can help you sleep like the Somnox 2 Sleep Robot. This 3-pound jellybean was developed by a Dutch inventor and you simply hold it against your chest like a teddy bear. Its soft, in-and-out movement encourages deep breathing. There's also the Dodow Sleep Aid, the Wesper Sleep Kit and the Casper Glow Light.

Tip #95: Dealing With Your Partner's Snoring

There's no feeling more intimate and secure than sleeping with your loved one. That's the good news. The bad news is that a partner can ruin your sleep. The big problem is if they snore, or they say that you snore. What can you do? First, sleep on your side and not your back. Today you can buy an adjustable bed base that will allow you to raise the head up so they (or you) stop snoring. Another option is to get an anti-snoring chin strap. This wraps around your head to keep your chin closed while you sleep. You might consider using a breathing strip on the nose to improve the air flow, which hopefully will reduce the volume of snoring. There's also mouth tape to keep your mouth closed. There are also devices that fit into the mouth to stop snoring like SnoreRX, ZQuiet and Pure Sleep.

Tip #96: What If It's More Than Snoring?

You're right, snoring may simply be a symptom of a much more serious problem called Sleep Apnea, and as many as 80% of the folks with it don't realize that they have it. People with Sleep Apnea make periodic gasping sounds along with their snoring as they stop breathing momentarily, which obviously interrupts their sleep. They may also feel very tired during the day because they don't sleep well. However not everyone with Sleep Apnea snores. There are actually three different types of Sleep Apnea beginning with Obstructive Sleep Apnea, which is the most common and it occurs when the throat muscles relax. Central Sleep Apnea occurs when the brain just doesn't send the proper signals to the muscles that control breathing. Last is Complex Sleep Apnea Syndrome, which is when someone has both Obstructive and Central Sleep Apnea. Yes, you probably want to see a doctor for a proper diagnosis of this condition, because it can be fatal.

Surgery is one way to correct the problem. Fortunately, there is another solution for this very serious problem called a Continuous Positive Airway Pressure machine or CPAP. There are a wide variety of styles and types of CPAP machines available, so you can find the one that works best for you, and your partner. They range from small travel-sized units to ones with heated airways to those with adjustable pressure. They all require a doctor's prescription but health insurance will help with the cost.

Tip #97: My Partner Is Kicking And Moving All Night

Restless Legs Syndrome, or Willis-Ekbom disease, is probably the most common condition you've never heard of before. RLS is estimated to affect up to 10% of the population and usually worsens with age. It is an unpleasant sensations in the legs described as burning or creeping, with an uncontrollable need to move them when at rest usually, beginning late in the day and evening. More than 80% of the people with RLS also have Periodic Limb Movement of Sleep or PLMS, which is the jerking or twitching of the legs during sleep every 15 to 40 seconds.

You may want to start treating these conditions with iron, magnesium or vitamin D supplements, all of which have been associated with improvements. A warm bath right before bed may also help you sleep better. Yes, movement also helps reduce the sensations, at least up until bedtime.

There are four FDA approved drugs to treat RLS including Requip, Mirapex, Horizant and Neupro. There are also drugs used off-label like Sinemet and Carbadopa/Levadopa. If you think you have RLS or PLMS you should contact an RLS treatment center.

Tip # 98: My Sleeping Partner Has Four Feet and Fur

Many pet owners enjoy having their pets sleep with them in the bed. In fact, I know dog owners who crate-trained their puppies only to decide to let them on the bed when they grew up. None of us want to sleep alone and our pets are part of our family, so it's only natural to want them with us at night. Studies have shown that sleeping with dogs is actually good for you by increasing security, reducing loneliness, easing insomnia and improving sleep quality. However dog and people sleep cycles are different, so there will be conflicts during the night so it's up to you to decide if it's worth it. Perhaps being in the bedroom is enough, maybe they don't really need to be on the bed with you.

Tip #99: I Wake Up With Sore Jaw Muscles

Sounds like you have a condition called bruxism or teeth grinding. This is caused by clenching your jaw muscles at night, which can lead to problems like headaches, jaw pain, even chipped teeth and sleep apnea. You can solve this problem and get better sleep with a mouth guard. There are three basic varieties. First is the custom impression mouth guard, which usually means a trip to your dentist. The second option is a boil-and-bite mouthguard that's made from a material that softens in hot water and then is allowed to cool so you can bite down on it. The last variety is a stock version or "one size fits all," which cannot be customized but are the least expensive choice.

Tip #100: My Friend Is Tired All the Time. Could It Be Narcolepsy?

Narcolepsy is very rare, only affecting about 50 people out of 100,000, but it is recognized by overwhelming daytime sleepiness and sudden attacks of sleep. Folks with it often have a hard time staying awake for long periods of time. Unfortunately it's a chronic condition without a cure, but medications can help manage the symptoms.

Tip #101: If I Get To Sleep, What Kind of Alarm Clock Should I Use?

There is almost every conceivable type of alarm clock available to help you get up on schedule. While some folks just use the alarm function on their cell phones, it's not the best idea. The blue light emitted by smartphones apparently makes it more difficult to fall asleep and stay asleep. Also having your phone near the bed makes it much easier for you to grab it to check your emails instead of sleeping. In other words, a stand-alone alarm clock may be your better choice and those that awaken you by increasing the ambient light like a natural sunrise are the best option. A sunrise alarm clock provides 30 to 40 minutes of gradually increasing light that mimics a sunrise. Whether you work the 2nd or 3rd shift, suffer from jet lag or just have to deal with insomnia, these dawn simulation alarm clocks are designed to wake you up gently and naturally. Many models also have features to help you fall asleep at night. While normal, old-fashioned alarm clocks wake you up with a jarring alarm sound that raises the cortisol levels in your body, these new sunrise alarm clocks wake you up naturally, which can also be effective in treating seasonal depression.

Sweet Dreams!

Your physical and mental health depends on getting a regular good night's sleep. Hopefully, these 101 tips will help you find what works for you to enjoy a wonderful night of sleep so you can wake up rested and refreshed. But you are a unique individual, so your best sleep will be unique, too. You have a unique set of genes and a unique set of epigenetics that impacts those genes. Your job, your family, your relationships, your health are just a few of the factors that make you, you. To optimize your life, you need good sleep every night, so you need to find out what works best for you. If these tips aren't enough, perhaps you need to check with your doctor of therapist to investigate what can be done to improve your sleep.

However, if none of these helps, you you're going to have to look at the other side of the equation, your work. Remember that your individual sleep pattern is based upon who you are, so if you're unable to find how to get a good night's sleep then it's time to change your work. If by nature you're a night owl then certainly a job at a dairy farm is a bad idea since they start work at 4 a.m. every day. If you're normally a morning person then a job as a night watchman or late-night DJ is a bad idea. You'll need to find a job that matches your genetic sleep pattern in one way or another in order to match your sleep cycle with your work.

Whatever it takes, I hope you find a great night's sleep!

About the Author

In my late 20s I began to have pain in my legs as if I'd run a marathon every day. It got so bad that I couldn't walk across our local mall without having to sit down and rest. I went to a range of doctors but nobody had any answers. One neurologist thought it must be psychosomatic but agreed to do a muscle biopsy in my left thigh, probably hoping to prove it was psychosomatic. He was shocked to discover that my muscle showed signs of damage at the cellular level, probably from overuse, but he didn't know why or what to do about it.

A few years later I woke up one morning feeling rested and realized that my legs didn't hurt. SLEEP! *That* was the problem. I quickly looked in the yellow pages (yes, this was many years ago) and there were two doctors listed under the sleep category. I called one and immediately made an appointment. This doctor suggested a sleep study and I quickly agreed.

The sleep study was simply getting wired up to a bunch of monitors overnight at his sleep lab, which was in the basement of the hospital. The following morning he asked me how I'd slept and I said it was the best night's sleep I'd had in months since it was a totally dark and quiet room. He then showed me a sample of a normal sleep pattern with its normal range of activity. Then he showed me my monitoring pattern. They didn't look anything alike. Mine looked like it was from someone running a race, which in fact, I had been. The doctor said I clearly had a bad case of Restless Legs Syndrome. I finally had a name for my sleep problem!

The good news was that there were drugs to help quiet my muscles while I slept and they were effective. The bad news is that none of them lasted forever. Most were effective for about 8 years before I had to change to another class of drugs. Today I anxiously await some new wonder drug so I can return to sleeping well at night.

Index

Your health is your greatest possession in this life so it's smart to look for the best ways to maintain and restore it as you age. In this guide you'll find treatments and therapies designed for your body and proven effective over decades, hundreds, even thousands of years. While not every therapy will work for every person, you can find the one that you need now or in the future in these pages. Take responsibility for your health right now, it's the only body you have, and read this book!

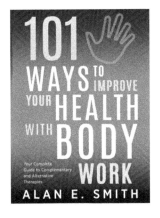

- Most comprehensive collection of body therapies available.

- Quick, easy-to-read descriptions of each treatment.

- Websites to learn more about each listing.

- Many subjects offer podcast listings featuring leading authorities.

- Find the most ancient to the most modern therapies.

- Rediscover the joy and beauty of living.

"Alan Smith's *Unbreak Your Health series* provides a terrific resource for those interested in real health!" --C. Norman Shealy, M.D., Ph.D.

"Knowledge is power. And this book is a way to provide you with a one stop source for discovering complementary and alternative therapies." --HealthStatus.com

"Five Stars --- Impressively organized and presented." --Midwest Book Review

Learn more at www.UnBreakYourHealth.com

Health & Fitness: Alternative Therapies

Find better health with your map to the world of complementary and alternative therapies in this comprehensive health and wellness guide for mind, body, and spirit.

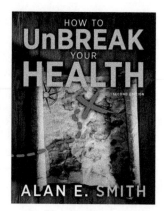

Are you sinking into the Quicksand of Pain? Are you stranded in the Mountains of Misery or simply lost in a Forest of Symptoms? Find your way to Hope with the 2nd edition of the award-winning book *How To UnBreak Your Health: Your Map to the World of Complementary and Alternative Therapies*. Discover how your body, mind and energy/spirit can work together to produce better health. Learn how to take charge of your health and find your path to the best health possible.

Trying to figure out where you are with your health problems, where you need to go and the best way to get there? You need a map to find your way around the amazing world of complementary or alternative therapies! Which therapies are right for you and your health problems? Find out in this easy-to-read guide to all of the therapies available outside the drugs-and-surgery world of mainstream medicine. Uncover the latest scientific research that's opening the door to therapies both ancient and modern that are available to help you improve your health.

- Discover health opportunities from Acupuncture to Zen Bodytherapy.
- Find out about the health benefits of Pilates, Yoga, and Massage.
- Learn about devices from Edgar Cayce's Radiac to the newest cold lasers.
- Hear from real people who've experienced these therapies and products.
- Locate free podcasts on the therapies you want to learn more about.

Learn more at www.UnBreakYourHealth.com

Health & Fitness: Alternative Therapies

CPSIA information can be obtained
at www.ICGtesting.com
Printed in the USA
BVHW012128210123
656729BV00039B/2275